DASH Diet Cookbook

Easy and Delicious Dash Diet Recipes

Disclaimer and Terms of Use:

Effort has been made to ensure that the
information in this book is accurate and
complete, however, the author and the
publisher do not warrant the accuracy of the
information, text and graphics contained within
the book due to the rapidly changing nature of
science, research, known and unknown facts
and internet. The Author and the publisher do
not hold any responsibility for errors,
omissions or contrary interpretation of the
subject matter herein. This book is presented
solely for motivational and informational
purposes only.

Contents

Table of Contents

Introduction

DASH stands for Dietary Approaches to Stop Hypertension.

It was created as a way to lower high blood pressure via a healthy diet.

The DASH diet has a whole range of health benefits though as it:
1. Reduces salt intake
2. Increases nutrient intake
3. Cuts out processed food
4. Reduces saturated fat, trans fats and cholesterol intake
5. Limits red meat
6. Limits added sugars
7. Promotes exercise
8. Helps you feel fuller for longer

It is beneficial for:
1. High blood pressure
2. Cancer prevention
3. Heart disease
4. Stroke prevention
5. Immune system
6. Diabetes
7. Osteoporosis prevention
8. Boosting energy levels
9. Weight loss

This chart shows the daily and weekly intakes of all the food groups, allowing you to create a weekly meal plan based around the recipes in the rest of this report.

WHOLEGRAINS	6-8 servings Daily	1oz dry cereal 1 slice wholemeal bread ½ cup cooked brown or wild rice ½ cup cooked whole wheat pasta ½ cup cooked whole wheat couscous 2 cups popcorn ½ cup sweet potato
VEGETABLES	4-5 servings Daily	½ cup of juice 1 cup raw ½ cup cooked
FRUITS	4-5 servings Daily	½ cup juice 1 cup raw ½ cup cooked 1 medium fruit ¼ cup dried
DAIRY	2-3 servings Daily	8oz milk Cup of yogurt 1 ½ oz cheese
LEAN PROTEINS	6oz or less Daily	1 egg 3 oz cooked lean meat 3 oz cooked

		poultry 3 oz cooked fish 3 oz tofu
NUTS, SEEDS, LEGUMES	4-5 servings Weekly	1 cup cooked legumes 1 ½ oz nuts 2 tbsp peanut butter 2 tbsp seeds
FATS AND OILS	2-3 servings Daily	1 tbsp mayonnaise 1 tbsp salad dressing 1 tsp oil 1 tsp butter
SWEETS	5 servings max Weekly	1 tbsp sugar 1 tbsp jam 1 cup lemonade
ALCOHOL	1 serving max (women) Daily 2 servings max (men) Daily At least 2 days of no alcohol a week	12 oz beer 5 oz wine 1.5 oz spirits

Breakfast Recipes

Homemade Muesli

Serves: 8

Ingredients

3 cups rolled oats
1 cup dried cranberries
1 cup raisins
1 cup sunflower seeds

Method

1. Mix all the ingredients together and stir in an airtight container.
2. Serve with 1 cup of skimmed milk or natural yogurt, a sprinkle of cinnamon and a portion of sliced, fresh fruit.

Melon, Cucumber and Grape Smoothie

Serves: 2

Ingredients

2 cups chopped cantaloupe melon
1 cup chopped cucumber
1 cup green grapes
2 cups yogurt

Method

1. Blend all the ingredients together until smooth.

Whole Wheat Blueberry Pancakes

Serves: 4

Ingredients

1 ¾ cup whole wheat self-raising flour
1 egg
1 ⅓ cup skimmed milk
1 cup blueberries
2 tbsp olive oil

Method
1. Whisk together the flour, egg and milk.
2. Stir the berries in.
3. Heat the oil in a frying pan and add 4 spoonfuls of the batter to the pan at a time. Press down on it slightly so they're about 3in diameter.
4. Cook for 2-3 minutes until the underneath is set and golden then flip them over and cook for a further 2-3 minutes until the bottom is browned.

Yogurt with Strawberries and Lime

Serves: 1

Ingredients

1 cup strawberries
Sprig of fresh mint
1 cup low fat natural yogurt
1 tsp vanilla extract
1 lime

Method

1. Roughly chop the strawberries and finely chop the mint and stir into the yogurt along with the vanilla.
2. Squeeze in the juice of ¼ of the lime.

Root Vegetable Hash topped with Poached Eggs

Serves: 4

Ingredients

½ cup diced parsnips
½ cup diced turnips
½ cup diced carrots
½ cup diced beetroot
½ cup diced sweet potatoes
½ cup diced swede
½ cup chunky diced apples
2tbsp parsley
4 tbsp olive oil
4 eggs

Method
1. Preheat the oven to 400 F (200 C).
2. Put the fruit and vegetables in a large roasting tin and sprinkle on the parsley. Drizzle over the oil and stir everything together.
3. Roast for 45-60 minutes until soft and golden brown. Stir them to turn every 15 minutes.
4. Boil a large pan of water.
5. Use a wooden spoon to make a whirlpool in the pan and break the eggs carefully into the water.
6. Cook for 4 minutes and remove with a slotted spoon. Drain on kitchen paper.
7. Plate up the roast mix and top with an egg, serve immediately.

Mini Feta Frittatas

Makes: 12

Ingredients
1 cup chopped onion
1 tbsp olive oil
2 cups chopped spinach
⅔ feta cheese
Cooking spray
6 eggs
100ml skimmed milk

Method

1. Preheat the oven to 375 F (190 C).
2. Heat the oil and cook the onion for 4-6 minutes until soft, stirring occasionally. Add the spinach for 2 minutes.
3. Cut the feta into small pieces and stir into the pan.
4. Whisk the eggs and milk together.
5. Grease a 12 hole muffin tin with the cooking spray and share out the cooked mixture between the holes.
6. Whisk together the eggs and milk and pour over the cooked mixture.
7. Bake for 20-25 minutes, until golden and cooked through.

Bruschetta topped with Apple Salsa

Serves: 1

Ingredients

2 x 1cm thick slices wholemeal baguette
½ red apple
½ small red onion
2 tomatoes
¼ red pepper
Sprig fresh coriander
¼ lime juice

Method

1. Put the baguette under a medium grill and toast both sides.
2. Finely chop all the ingredients, except the lime, and mix together with the lime juice.
3. Top the bread with the salsa.

Lunch Recipes

Salmon Fishcakes with Grapefruit Salad

Serves: 2

Ingredients

½ cooked petit pois
½ cup grapefruit segments
1 cup basil leaves
1 cup spinach leaves
½ sliced red onion
2 tbsp balsamic vinegar

1 cup chopped sweet potatoes
6oz tinned salmon fillet, in water
1 clove garlic
½ bunch of spring onions
¼ red chilli
½ tsp dried coriander
Slice white bread
2 tbsp plain flour
1 egg, beaten

Method

1. Boil the potatoes for 20 minutes until tender then mash until lump free.
2. Blend the garlic, chili and spring onions and mix with the fish and potatoes. Use a little of the tin water to bind it if necessary.

3. Shape into 2 cakes then chill for 1 hour.
4. Preheat the oven to 400 F (200 C).
5. Blend the bread until it is fine breadcrumbs.
6. Dip the cakes first into the flour, then the egg and finally the breadcrumbs. Bake for 20-25 minutes until golden brown and cooked through.

Mushroom and Aubergine Burgers in Whole Wheat Brioche Buns

Serves: 2

Ingredients

25g margarine
300g whole wheat flour
1 tsp sugar
1 pack fast action yeast
100ml milk
50ml water
1 beaten egg

2 portobello mushrooms
2 thick slices eggplant
1 tbsp olive oil
2 thick slices from beef tomatoes

Method

1. Rub the margarine into the flour then add the sugar and yeast.
2. Add the wet ingredients and knead for 10 minutes.
3. Cover and leave in a warm place for 1 ½ hours to double in size.
4. Knead for another 5 minutes then shape into 2 burger buns and leave for a further hour.
5. Preheat the oven to 400 F (200 C). Bake the buns for 20-25 minutes until they are cooked through.

6. Brush the mushrooms and eggplant with the oil then roast for 10 minutes, turn over and cook for a further 5 minutes until soft.
7. Stack a cooked mushroom and eggplant slice in a brioche bun along with a slice of tomato and serve immediately.

Chicken Noodle Soup

Serves: 2

Ingredients

½ onion, diced
1 tbsp olive oil
3 cups low sodium chicken broth
Juice of 1 lemon
½ cup chopped carrots
2 cups whole wheat spaghetti, broken into inch long pieces
6oz cooked chicken breast
1 tbsp chopped parsley
½ cup frozen sweetcorn

Method
1. Soften the onion in the oil for 5 minutes.
2. Add the broth and lemon juice and bring to the boil.
3. Add the carrots and simmer for 10 minutes, until tender.
4. Stir the spaghetti in for 5 minutes, until soft.
5. Add the chicken, parsley and sweetcorn for 5 minutes, until heated through and serve immediately.

Vegetable Packed Macaroni Cheese

Serves: 2

Ingredients

1 tbsp low fat margarine
1 tbsp flour
8oz skimmed milk
½ oz grated low fat cheddar
½ oz grated parmesan
1 tsp nutmeg

½ cup cauliflower florets
½ sliced leeks
2 minced garlic cloves
1 tsp margarine
½ cup frozen sweetcorn
½ cup cherry tomatoes

Method

1. Preheat the oven to 375 F (190 C).
2. Melt the tbsp margarine in a large sauce pan and stir in the flour to a smooth paste. Gradually whisk in the milk, making sure the sauce is smooth and lump free between additions. Stir in the cheese and nutmeg until the cheese has melted.
3. Boil the cauliflower for 5 minutes.
4. Melt the tsp margarine and soften the leeks and garlic for 5 minutes.
5. Stir the leeks, corn and tomatoes into the cheese sauce and pour into a roasting dish.
6. Bake for 15-20 minutes until browned on the top.

Tuna and Mixed Bean Salad

Serves: 2

Ingredients

2 tsp olive oil
1 tbsp red wine vinegar
1 clove minced garlic

½ cup cherry tomatoes
½ cup cooked green beans
½ cup rocket
½ sliced red onion
¼ cucumber, diced

1 tin of tuna, in water
1 tin of mixed beans, rinsed
2 boiled eggs, cut into wedges

Method

1. Whisk together the oil, vinegar and garlic.
2. Mix together the salad vegetables. Add the tuna, beans and eggs.
3. Serve the salad and drizzle over the dressing.

Leek and Potato Soup

Serves: 2

Ingredients

½ sliced onion
1 cup sliced leeks
1 tbsp margarine
2 cups chicken broth
1 bay leaf
1 cup diced potato
½ cup natural yogurt
1 tbsp chives

Method
1. Cook the onion and leeks in the margarine for 5 minutes until soft.
2. Add the broth and bay leaf and cook for 5 minutes.
3. Add the potatoes, boil then simmer for 20-25 minutes until tender.
4. Remove the bay leaf and blend with the yogurt. Return to the pan, with the chives, and heat through for 2-3 minutes. Serve immediately.

Simple Tomato and Pesto Pasta

Serves: 2

Ingredients

1 cup uncooked pasta, any shape

Small handful of basil
3oz parmesan cheese
1 garlic clove
5 tbsp olive oil

1 clove minced garlic
½ red chili, minced
2 tsp olive oil
1 tin chopped tomatoes

Method
1. Cook the pasta according to the packet instructions.
2. Blend the basil, cheese, 1 garlic clove and 5 tbsp oil until smooth.
3. Cook the garlic and chili in the oil for 3-5 minutes until beginning to brown, add the tomatoes.
4. Stir the pasta into the tomato sauce and cook for a further 3 minutes until it's coated.
5. Serve the pasta into bowls and drizzle over some of the pesto.
6. Chill the remaining pesto and save it for up to 3 weeks to add to any other dish.

Dinner Recipes

Roasted Vegetable Lasagne

Serves: 4

Ingredients

2 peppers
1 red onion
2 zucchini
1 eggplant
2 tbsp olive oil

2 tbsp low fat margarine
2 tbsp flour
16oz skimmed milk
3oz grated low fat cheddar
3oz grated parmesan
1 tsp nutmeg

1 cup cherry tomatoes
Handful fresh basil
2 tins chopped tomatoes
160g whole wheat lasagne sheets
Dried oregano

Method

1. Preheat the oven to 400 F (200 C).
2. Cut the peppers, onion, zucchini and egg
   medium sized chunks and toss in the oil. Roast

in a large, deep sided dish for 15-25 minutes until soft and just beginning to brown.

3. Melt the margarine in a large sauce pan and stir in the flour to a smooth paste. Gradually whisk in the milk, making sure the sauce is smooth and lump free between additions. Stir in the cheese and nutmeg until the cheese has melted.
4. Halve the cherry tomatoes and chop the basil.
5. Remove the vegetables from the oven and turn it down to 375 F (190 C).
6. Stir the tinned tomatoes and basil into the vegetables then top them with the lasagne sheets.
7. Pour over the cheese sauce, dot the surface with the tomatoes and sprinkle over some oregano. Bake for 40-50 minutes until golden brown.

Pitta Pizza

Serves: 2

Ingredients

2 wholemeal pitta breads
1 ½ oz mozzarella
2 tbsp tomato paste
½ cup mushrooms
½ cup red onions
½ cup olives
½ cup peppers
1 jalapeno
3oz grated mozzarella
2 tsp oregano

Method

1. Preheat the oven to 375 F (190 C).
2. Spread the paste over the pittas.
3. Slice the vegetables and top the pittas with them, any leftover vegetables can be eaten raw as a salad.
4. Over the pizza with mozzarella and sprinkle over the oregano.
5. Cook for 8-10 minutes until piping hot and the cheese has melted.

Lentil, Chickpea and Sweet Potato Curry with Chapatti

Serves: 4

Ingredients

1 cup onions
2 cloves garlic
1 tbsp olive oil
2 tsp garam masala
2 tsp cumin seeds, dry-fried and ground
1 tsp chili powder (mild or hot)
1 tsp coriander seed, dry-fried and ground
1 cup red lentils
1 cup chickpeas
1 litre vegetable broth
2 tins chopped tomatoes
2 tbsp tomato purée
1 cup diced sweet potatoes

1 cup whole wheat flour
½ water

Method

1. Slice the onions and garlic and fry in the oil for 4-6 minutes until soft but not coloured.
2 Stir in the spices for 1 minute.
3 Add the rest of the ingredients and bring to the boil. Then cover and simmer for 20-25 minutes until everything is soft.
4 Knead the flour and water into a soft dough. Divide it into 4 balls then roll out as thin as possible.

5   Heat a skillet and dry fry one chapatti at a time
    for 1-2 minutes each side until both are
    blistered and golden brown.

Tomato Fish Pie

Serves: 4

Ingredients

1 cup diced onion
1 tbsp olive oil
1 cup chopped kale
2 tsp parsley
2 tsp tarragon
3 tins chopped tomatoes
Tbsp tomato paste
8oz salmon
2 cups sliced sweet potato

3 cups frozen petit pois
1 tsp parsley
½ lemon juice

Method
1. Heat the oil in a large saucepan and cook the onion for 4-5 minutes until soft and beginning to colour. Add the kale for 5 minutes, until wilted.
2. Add the herbs and then the tomatoes and paste. Bring to the boil then add the fish and simmer for 15 minutes.
3. Preheat the oven to 400 F (200 C).
4. Transfer the fish and tomato mixture to an ovenproof dish and top with the slices of potato. Bake for 35-45 minutes until the potatoes are going crispy round the edges.
5. Cook the peas according to the packet instructions. Drain and mash with the parsley and lemon juice.

Paella

Serves: 4

Ingredients

2 tbsp olive oil
4 cloves garlic
2 tsp paprika
1 cup diced red onion
1 cup chopped green peppers
6oz chicken breast, skin off
2 tsp thyme
2 cups uncooked brown or wild rice
2 tins chopped tomatoes
700ml low sodium chicken stock
2oz cooked prawns

Method
1. Crush the garlic cloves and dice the chicken.
2. Heat the oil in a large saucepan and fry the garlic, paprika, onion, peppers and chicken for 5-10 minutes, until the chicken is coloured all over.
3. Add the thyme and the rice; stir well to coat the rice in oil.
4. Add the tomatoes and stock and simmer for 15-25 minutes until the sauce is beginning to thicken.
5. Add the prawns for the last 5 minutes cooking time.

Tofu Stir Fry

Serves: 4

Ingredients

2 cups uncooked brown or wild rice
4 cloves garlic
12oz firm tofu
2 tbsp olive oil
2 the ground ginger
½ tsp 5 spice powder
2 tbsp corn starch
1 cup raw carrots
1 cup mushrooms
1 cup broccoli florets
1 cup bean sprouts
2 tsp sesame oil

Method

1. Cook the rice according to the packet instructions.
2. Thin slice the garlic.
3. Marinate the tofu in the olive oil, garlic, ginger and 5 spice powder for at least 30 minutes.
4. Thin slice the carrots and mushrooms.
5. Remove the tofu from the marinade and put in a bowl with the corn starch, keep the marinade for the next step. Toss to coat it.
6. Heat half of the marinade in a medium pan and cook the tofu for 5-6 minutes, until brown all over, stirring it gently.
7. Heat the other half of the marinade in a wok and cook the vegetables until the tofu is done.

Add 2 tsp of sesame at the end of cooking and stir the tofu in to combine everything.

8. Serve immediately.

Turkey Pastitsio

Serves: 4

Ingredients

2 cups whole wheat pasta, any shape
1 cup onions
2 cloves garlic
1 tbsp olive oil
12oz turkey mince
1 eggplant
2 tsp cinnamon
2 tsp oregano
1 tin chopped tomatoes
200ml chicken broth

2 tbsp low fat margarine
2 tbsp flour
16oz skimmed milk
3oz grated low fat cheddar
3oz grated parmesan
1 tsp nutmeg

Method

1. Preheat the oven to 400 F (200 C).
2. Cook the pasta according to packet instructions.
3. Slice the onions and garlic and fry in the oil for 5 minutes until soft.
4. Add the meat for 10-12 minutes until brown throughout.
5. Dice the eggplant and add to the meat along with the cinnamon, oregano, tomatoes and

broth. Bring to the boil then simmer for 30 minutes.

6. Melt the margarine in a large sauce pan and stir in the flour to a smooth paste. Gradually whisk in the milk, making sure the sauce is smooth and lump free between additions. Stir in the cheese and nutmeg until the cheese has melted.

7. Mix the pasta into the meat sauce and tip into an ovenproof serving dish, top with the cheese sauce and bake for 35-40 minutes until golden brown on top.

Vanilla and Raisin Rice Pudding

Serves: 4

Ingredients

1 cup uncooked brown rice
4 cups skimmed milk
2 tsp vanilla extract
1 tbsp soft brown sugar
I tbsp honey
1 cup raisins

Method
1. Cook the rice according to the packet instructions until the liquid has been absorbed.
2. Add the milk, vanilla and sugar to the pan, bring to the boil then simmer for 15 minutes, stirring regularly.
3. Add the honey and raisins for a further 15 minutes, still stirring.
4. Serve while hot.

Cinnamon Popcorn

Serves: 1

Ingredients

⅛ tsp cinnamon
1 tsp caster sugar
2 tsp olive oil
1 tbsp unpopped popcorn

Method

1. Mix the cinnamon and sugar together.
2. Heat the oil in a large, lidded pan. Add the corn and give it a shake. Put the lid on.
3. When the corn begins to pop, shake the pan until the popping slows, then pour into a serving bowl.
4. Sprinkle on the cinnamon sugar, immediately.

Flapjack

Makes: 12

Ingredients

3 bananas
1 apple
3 tbsp low fat margarine
2 tbsp peanut butter
3 tbsp honey
3 cups rolled oats
2 cups dried apricots
2 tsp ground ginger

Method

1. Preheat oven to 325 F (170 C).
2. Mash the bananas and peel and chop the apple.
3. Melt the margarine, butter and honey in a pan, add the apple and banana as well as ½ cup water then tip it all into a large, heatproof bowl.
4. Add the oats, apricot and ginger to the bowl and mix well.
5. Tip the mixture into a square, greased and lined baking dish and spread it out.
6. Bake for 50-60 minutes until golden brown on the top.
7. Cool in the tin before cutting into portions.

Beetroot and Apple Bran Muffins

Makes: 6

Ingredients

1 tbsp low fat margarine
⅔ cup of self-raising flour
1 tsp cinnamon
1 tbsp soft brown sugar
¼ cup skimmed milk
1 tsp vanilla extract
½ cup unsweetened apple juice
2 apples
3 tbsp bran flakes
⅓ cup grated beetroot

Method

1. Preheat the oven to 350 F (180 C).
2. Melt the margarine.
3. Sift the flour and cinnamon into a bowl and add the sugar. Stir in the milk, vanilla and juice.
4. Peel the apples and finely chop, then stir into the cake mix.
5. Add the cereal and leave it for five minutes.
6. Stir the beetroot in and make sure it all thoroughly mixed.
7. Put into 6 muffin cases and bake for 20-25 minutes until golden brown.
8. Cool in the tin before removing.

Conclusion

This book is the start of the new you. Following these recipes should put you on the right path, direct to good health. Build up your new regime slowly to ensure future success and gradually add exercise to your daily routine.

www.ingramcontent.com/pod-product-compliance
Lightning Source LLC
Chambersburg PA
CBHW060345290526
45791CB00004B/1535